Medical Writing for Smart People

Because dummies shouldn't write about medicine

Table of Contents

Acknowledgements

I was in a Los Angeles hotel elevator in town to film a series of interviews for a nationwide chronic obstructive pulmonary disease (COPD) drug launch. To access the club level you insert a special key. A child with another family exclaimed how she wished she could stay on the fancy higher floor. Another executive in the elevator leaned over saying:

"We have to spend a lot of time away from our families. They try to make us feel better by giving us grander hotel rooms and fancy amenities but we would rather be with our kids in a hotel, on a lower floor, on vacation."

Thank you to Steve, Harrison, and Ryland for joining me and making the journey better but mostly for the times when I left you behind. One evening we were watching a movie, Notting Hill. A visually stunning scene displays seasons passing in a montage of memories as Bill Withers sings, "Ain't No Sunshine When She's Gone"--my toddler son stated that the song reminds him of me when I have to get on an airplane--it was time to change my work life. I hope that you find useful insights for wherever you might be in your writing journey. And bring the sunshine along for the ride.

What exactly *is* a medical writer?

Even as a slightly active member of society you are certainly asked what you do for a living. I have trotted out a variety of responses over the years and the reactions range from glazed eyes to shades of genuine interest. More frequently I observe overall confusion. When feeling cheeky I will respond, "I am a writer." People get excited and ask about my publications. "Oh, would I perhaps have read any of your books?" Not being entirely well behaved I mention a popular series on hepatobiliary disease and let them sort it out. Once I was asked did I write the prescription information on pill bottles. I just mentioned that I couldn't write that small and left it at that. I don't live in a metropolitan city so I may be more of an oddity here south of the Mason-Dixon line.

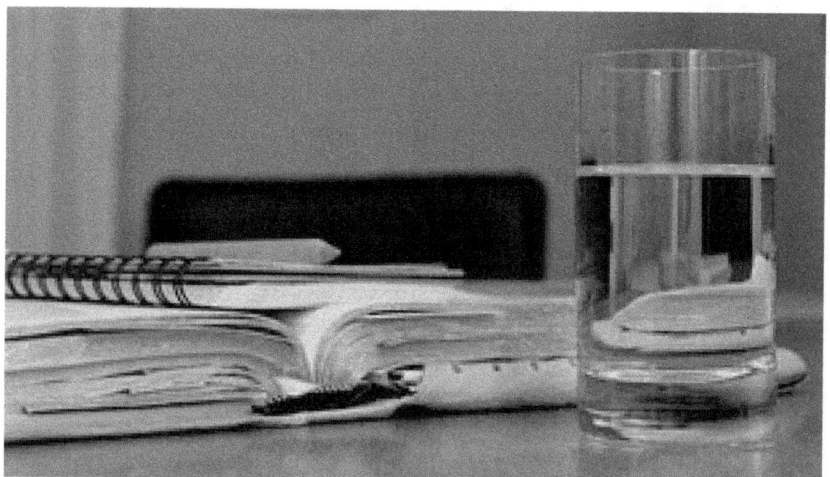

Writing professionally for almost 20 years, I appreciate the nuance of different aspects of medical writing. I define a medical writer as developing content about the practice of clinical medicine, clinical research, or the health policy and economics influencing decisions at the point of care. I distinguish the role of a scientific writer as being more directed toward a lay audience. Personally unable to claim success at nailing 8th-grade level a la Flesch-Kincaid writing, I stopped trying after a client asked me to describe a ureter based on its resemblance to spaghetti. And then I was subsequently fired for the apparent important lack of the marketable skill. Or when challenged to write National Institute of Health (NIH) Congressional Justifications for government funding informed the writing had to be 8th grade level or it couldn't go to congress for review. Yes. Really.

My original perspective for this book was along the lines of Anthony Bourdain in Kitchen Confidential--a raw, informative, but not always pretty account of the medical writer's daily life. Thinking of the repercussions of telling such a substantive story I recall an Anne Lamott quote,

"You own everything that happened to you. Tell your stories. If people wanted you to write warmly about them, they should have behaved better."

I decided to add a few anecdotes throughout but keep the overall vibe informative, authentic, and hopefully a bit insightful. A ton of books are already in the marketplace about writing with advice and step-by-step instruction describing how to improve skills, land clients, and walk off into the sunset with a rainbow over your head and a puppy frolicking at your heels. This isn't that book. I am an accidental medical writer--a little talent and a whole bunch of lightening in the right place at the right time. But I am convinced that some of it will bring value to either your consumer eye or your writing practice.

My educational background in the biological sciences and Chiropractic (doctorate) included studies in statistics, working with patients in a clinical environment, and conducting bench research (population genetics). Medical writing includes a wide open field for a variety of writers. Do you need advanced degrees or even any degree to write about science or medical topics? I am more inclined to think it depends on the type of writing and your desired audience (physician, academic, patient population, government). Are you able to craft a meaningful question? What does your audience need to hear? How will you structure information?

> **"Writing is not a special language owned by the English teacher. Writing is thinking on paper. Anyone who thinks clearly can write clearly, about anything at all. Science, demystified, is just another nonfiction subject. Writing, demystified, is just another way for scientists to transmit what they know."--On Writing Well by William Zinsser**

I think a Master of Science (MSc) academic post-graduate degree provides the structure of developing a research project, analyzing data, and writing up a scientific thesis relevant to critical thinking and communication. Quite often PhDs are preferred but in my case I don't know what an additional year of--*Constraints of Landscape Pattern and Fish Mobility on Ecological Genetics of Lake (Salvelinus namaycush) and Arctic Char (Salvelinus alpine) in Arctic Watersheds* rigorous study would have contributed to my insights as a medical writer. Over the span of several years I worked in labs where we developed a method for extracting DNA from outdated ethanol samples, mixed taq polymerase, learned how to run a DNA sequence machine, pipetted myself cross-eyed, saved samples from catastrophe in the minus 70 degree freezer, applied (and analyzed) an appropriate mutation model for DNA microsatellites, wrote a well-received thesis and personally went home with more than my share of mutated drosophila melanogaster hitchhikers in my long, densely, curly hair.

There really isn't a perfect pedigree. The ability to distill complicated medical and statistical information into concise, accurate, and compelling narrative is the goal but often hiring the right person for the job gets lost in the degree. There are lousy writers of all stripes. Your mileage may vary.

You can't please everyone, you aren't a pizza

The American Medical Writer's Association has free introductory information about becoming a medical writer. Here are a few types of projects listed on the website. Look them up especially if exploring opportunities or new to the field.

-Abstracts and posters for medical conferences

-Advertising copy for pharmaceuticals and other products

-Advisory board summaries

-Books

-Editing (including substantive editing, proofreading, and fact checking)

-Journal abstracts

-Managed market training

-Medical education materials, including continuing medical education needs assessments and programs, physician and medical science liaison training, and patient education (including web-based interactive educational programs)

-Monographs

-Multimedia projects

-Pharmaceutical marketing and advertising

-Physician speeches and presentations

-Practice management materials

-Proposal writing

-Regulatory documents (including clinical trial reports, Common Technical Documentation, integrated summaries of efficacy and safety, investigator brochures, Investigational New Drug documents, New Drug Application submissions, protocols)

-Sales training materials including e-learning modules

-Slide presentations and kits

-Scripts for DVD and other multimedia and Web-based formats

-Web content

-White paper

So now what?

I launched my official medical writing career in big pharma writing clinical study protocols and other regulatory documents associated with launching drugs targeting human immunodeficiency virus (HIV). The golden age of industry included American Express gift cards for working a little extra or company wide celebrations and incentivized after hour celebrations. For me, regulatory writing was an appropriate place to learn the "nuts and bolts" of clinical writing. There is no room for narrative voice or highly stylized writing as specific guidance documents dictate development of content. If regulatory writing is your focus, ample resources abound--just a Google search away. After a one-year contract I transitioned my pregnancy leave into a hiatus in the aftermath of a "friendly" merger more akin to a hostile takeover. Colleagues and co-workers were unceremoniously escorted out of their cubicles without notice while many senior executives exited with severance and opportunities earmarked as they sped out of parking lots.

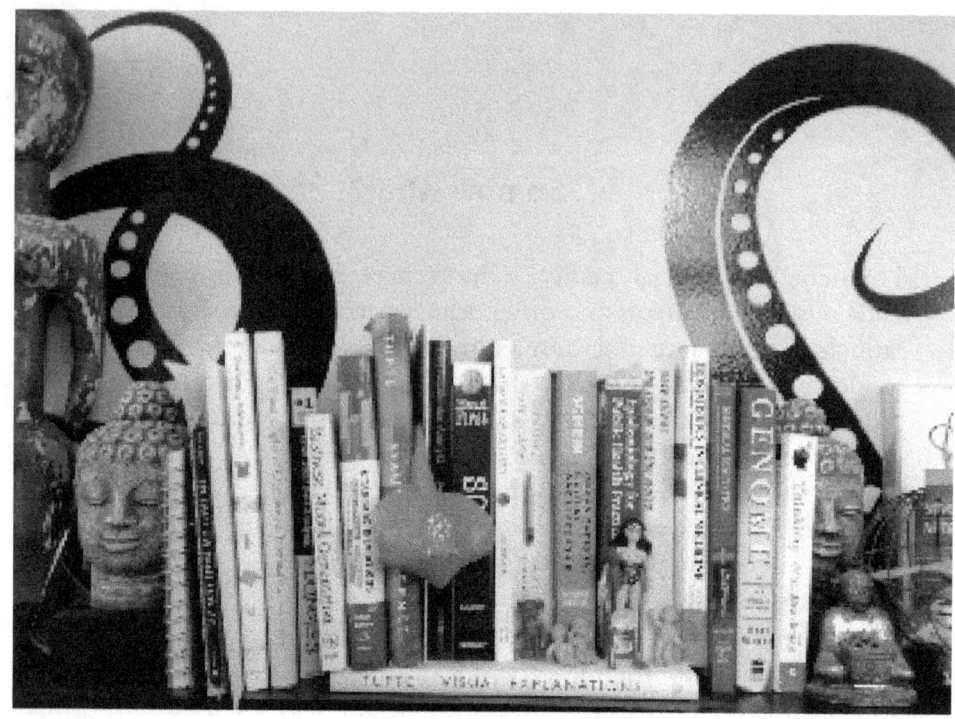

Biotechnology companies started popping up in the wake of the industry diaspora. Opportunities to collaborate with key industry opinion leaders followed. A former colleague called for help writing an infectious disease manuscript and puzzled by the rather large compensation I happily accepted. Dear reader, I was hooked. The opportunity to research a variety of topics and write articles is mesmerizing. Just when you might experience boredom another new and exciting medical advance claims your attention and expertise. I remember attending an industry meeting seated at the same table as a leading HIV research expert. I was tempted to introduce myself as the ghostwriter of his last review article but thought better of it. Manuscript writing can be a great source of income but the long timelines often delay compensation especially when relying on multiple reviews and ongoing meetings and revision. Modern day whiffs of bias and economic driven endpoints create a murky industry-sponsored document pipeline problematic if a reputable company or client base does not support you. Caveat emptor my friends.

In recent years I invested considerable time and resources developing data analytics skills. Strong statistical fluency helps avoid unwittingly introducing biased marketing objectives into your content development. One of my favorite quotes is **"In God we trust, all others bring data"** attributed to William Edwards Deming -- a renowned American statistician. I will repeat the battle cry of a good course in statistics throughout the book. Not only will your writing be infused with clarity and validity it helps to develop a keen research eye. Understanding how to distinguish meaningful evidence supporting clinical practice behavior is a nontrivial task of medical content development.

Don't let me sway you from pursuing a career in continuing medical education but I will provide a few cautionary tales. In my opinion, there are low-value agency practices fueled by greed and opportunities to land the next funded program. After all--it is a numbers game. Write a bunch of need assessments for proposals of dubious merit and eventually something is funded. In my "n of 1" experience, once the funding amount is confirmed the trimming of services begins. We had a saying, "*selling the dream and implementing the nightmare*". I have been writing for over 20 years and found myself unable to tolerate the whims and fancies of clients often unwilling to firewall the content from stakeholder content facilitators.

Don't get me wrong. There is a lot of meaningful work to be done. It can just be soul sucking at times. The biggest companies often have the most to lose so, how should I put this? They often cut the most corners. Brought in a total of 4 times to meet with hiring managers at one of the largest medical education companies I bristle at the low quality output I reviewed. At one 2-day interview the entire executive team was missing in action, another time provided with a poorly written report I was asked to outline an article based on the findings. Here is my email highlighting the deficiencies in the report...

> **"I have reviewed the report and created an outline for an article. There is a caveat as I did interpret the task from a value messaging perspective. Understandably when we prepare outcomes reports we publish and report summary statistics rolled up to a certain level so we can provide a snapshot of an activity and general trends in the**

data we have analyzed. The first outline is a general commentary on potential insights if there is an opportunity to optimize the data collection. Since I do not know what was presented in the activity I just wanted to give my mile high impressions. The second outline is for a specific article for the realistic scenario that we may have all of the analytics we are going to have so all things being equal where do I see the story. I hope that isn't too confusing or beyond the scope of

what you wanted to see. From a "value" perspective I would suggest that a higher level of granularity is needed. I know this may be risky as a candidate for a position I would very much like to fill but I also feel strongly that I must contribute the type of insights you can anticipate if I was indeed collaborating with a team. The data integrated into the report would need stratification by demographic factors as well as self-efficacy assessment responses to reveal the patterns and granularity in a different light than a summary

report might provide. For example, I would be interested in seeing primary care provider (PCP) and psychiatrist data on the same graphic—where

do they align? Where do they differ? Outliers? I would also be interested in seeing what patterns might be revealed if we stratify by patient load, self-efficacy assessment scores or other demographics. Quite often the compelling stories are hidden in the data and we just need to use a data strategy or a pivot analysis to dig a little deeper. Including a few additional demographic or clinical practice questions would also add richness to subsequent discussions, articles, or specifically targeted insights for future education. I included comments in the outline for your review and welcome the opportunity to clarify my impressions and suggestions."

Truly characteristic of this organization, after careful review of the data and wresting with the low quality of data generation and collection, I never heard a peep. Granted, the email is painful to read as I see now how I struggled with communicating the real story. There wasn't anything meaningful or robust to report. They allegedly hired internally for the position. I was surprised about the measures being collected in a medical education intervention. No questions about suicide ideation, how to manage transition of care, or social determinants--just specific drug prescribing. We can do better.

Developing a variety of writing skills will help provide diverse and ongoing opportunities. The little black dress of writing medical content is currently HEOR. Health economics and outcomes research (HEOR) has become de rigueur in evaluating quality assessments and meeting the growing evidentiary demand among healthcare industry stakeholders. What type of writing is needed in HEOR? The International Society of Pharmacoeconomics (ISPOR) provides guidance documents and many tools for conducting, understanding, or writing about outcomes research. Having the ability to distill medical knowledge clearly, familiarity or experience with research, organization skills, and writing aptitude are common skills for the general framework of a medical or scientific writer. Discussing clinical medicine without consideration of cost, value, or health policy in today's healthcare environment is like trying to stand on a two-legged stool.

HEOR writing distinguishes the "value" of innovation as novel therapies transition to the armatorium of available devices and treatments in the evolving healthcare marketplace. A skilled writer is needed to communicate the real-world value of treatments. No longer are we evaluating evidence-based care solely on randomized controlled trial results where patients are homogenized for extrapolation of well-controlled experimental findings. Real world data from efficacy and safety evaluations in the complex patient is relevant and critical for continued market access. Market decisions, professional society accountability, governance, and epidemiological analyses to improve experiential outcomes enhance available data to include real world evidence. Although HEOR is typically aligned with industry, this represents only a single application of outcomes research. A research question, conceptual model, variable identification, appropriate measure selection and analysis plans have broad applicability in many medical content scenarios. For example, I strive to represent an "outside in" approach to developing content. My niche involves business-to-business content media integrating context from health economics, health policy, and clinical research/medicine delivered directly to the healthcare provider or professional society.

Luckily the digital age provides opportunities to write about medicine in your own authentic voice. The ability to integrate discussions of economics and health policy into narratives of clinical medicine provides limitless possibilities. Developing a blog either for established platforms or developing a personal brand is big business. Copy writing, copy marketing, brand marketing, and just the art of storytelling continues to drive opportunities limited only by your imagination. Clients often need a narrative. Data collection is a primary focus of many healthcare organizations but often lacks answers to "now what or so what?" The storytelling or narrative engages and contextualizes why we should care about an innovation, therapy, or disease outcome. Developing marketing content where there is "permission" and a need can be informative. My practice is to let science lead the message. Unfortunately a parallel business model often emerges where marketing messages evolve first and a hunt for science to support the claims follow. Become astute at differentiating the two. Think about a brand in need of a marketing campaign. The ability to create context for industry white papers, position papers, or corporate blogs is in high demand. If you are in doubt, take a look at Open by American Express. A small business portal that at first glance isn't "selling" provides a dashboard with a library of tools and content. This is the heart of permission marketing. **Provide a service, create a tribe, and bring value.**

Don't limit opportunities unless you find a writing style uniquely your own that ticks all of the boxes. Jim Carrey said something in a commencement speech that was point on. He was talking about his father trading his dream of a career in comedy for a reliable consistent job as an accountant. After 12 years working for the same company his father was laid off. Jim learned an important lesson at a young age.

"You can fail at what you don't want, so you might as well do what you love."

Tools for writing

If resources are limited and you hope to start writing sooner rather than later I wouldn't worry about taking courses or certifications just yet. I have never heard anything unique about becoming a medical writer on either a webinar or in a workshop. The low hanging fruit has already been picked. Avoid the heavy peach and follow your interests. First of all, we have unique skills and learn differently. I am a visual learner while others need to disappear with a text to absorb anything. In this day and age of Coursera and other massive open online content (MOOC) you can learn from the best and customize courses to a "just in time" need, a specific project, or a future professional goal. Reading medical, pharmaceutical, and health economics journals are useful and informative. I subscribe to NEJM, JAMA, and other journals that send abstracts by email. I find the table of contents timely about what high-level topics are trending and relevant for further exploration.

Statistics courses for medicine and biostatistics will provide examples similar to what you might expect to see in your daily routine. Although not necessarily a book for the expert in the field of data visualization, Medical Illuminations by Howard Wainer refines best practices of displaying medical evidence accurately and in a compelling informative manner. The use of examples from the literature citing such pioneers as Edward Tufte and the origins of evidenced-based medicine by Pierre Charles Alexandre Louis's 1835 discrediting the efficacy of "bloodletting".

E A few data suggestions to keep in mind...

-To improve visibility, avoid light colors--don't assume access to color printing--include distinctive markings retained in black & white printing
-Label both ends of a graph (if lines are crossing) to avoid confusion
-Select appropriate spacing intervals for axes (be careful not to distort data)
-This is a pet peeve of mine--labels MUST be easily read and

positioned clearly

-When including a "Total" or an "All" label make it clearly distinct from other labels

-Use the x-axis label to clearly describe the display (it should be explicit)

-Data points should not sit on the axis--add appropriate spacing

-Remove extraneous plot points

-Pay attention to font selection--try something new to provide visual interest

Best practices from decades ago have evolved with the digital economy. Historically all we needed was an outline and the subsequent approval to begin drafting content. Armed with a subscription to a well-stocked medical library and current word processing software I possessed the necessary tools of the trade. Fast forward to now and my office is customized by client needs, able to manage proprietary data on security laptops, passports to attend international meetings, security access to data, clearance into NIH meetings, and dozens of industry and healthcare stakeholder conferences, meetings, private panel discussions and endless teleconferences across a variety of time zones. Think about the tools and resources that you rely on again and again. What do they have in common? Do you always use them the same way? A carefully edited professional library can be collected overtime and is a valuable resource for content development.

Here are my top ten books in random order.

-A Bittersweet Season Caring for Our Aging Parents—and Ourselves

-Mythologies by Roland Barthes

-The Lady Tasting Tea by David Salsburg

-Lapham's Quarterly Volume II, Number 4 Fall 2009 Medicine

-Thinking Fast and Slow by Daniel Kahneman

-The Visual Display of Quantitative Information by Edward Tufte

-Decision Modeling for Health Economic Evaluation by Briggs, Sculpher, and Claxton

-The Checklist Manifesto by Atul Gawande

-Medical Statistics: A Textbook for the Health Sciences by Machin, Campbell, Walters

-Genome: The Autobiography of a Species in 23 Chapters

Edit

Useful Tools...your mileage may vary

MacBook Pro: I realize not everyone ascribes to the religion of Apple but I am so happy in my rose-colored glasses that I can't see any of you.

iPad: Showing up with a laptop no matter how inconspicuous is a pain and gets in the way of engaging and being present. I tend to use the iPad and sync everything to the laptop once back in my hotel or in my home office. And think of the money you save by downloading a few movies to watch later instead of viewing hotel overpriced offerings.

iPhone: The camera function and audio have been upgraded and I find that I can get decent sound quality while on the road. I also rely on the mapping apps, podcasts, calendar, and Evernote to keep my office humming along from wherever I am. Android also has a variety of apps that improve efficiency.

Back-up charger for phone: If you attend conferences you must have been gifted one of these and they are spectacular. If not, be on the hunt.

Digital voice recorder: I loved my old Olympus but alas it doesn't talk the language of Apple so I am in the market for an upgrade. A digital recorder is useful in briefings to capture the narrative and has high enough quality to record sound from the middle of the room.

Last but not least is a projector. Yes. You heard me right. Clearly not a "need" but boy it sure is convenient. I can't tell you how many times a projector has saved the day. One advantage to the Apple integration is that I just plug it directly into my iPhone, iPad, or laptop and BOOM I am sharing high quality images on the wall of a hotel room or for the faint of heart, an actual screen. There are small mobile models that integrate readily with your preferred computer.

I love my blue yeti for conference calls, podcasts, or just high quality Skype calls that I might want to record and integrate into my website down the road. It is important to have a tool for decent sound quality especially if like me you work remotely. You don't want to sound like you are sitting in a windowless bathroom.

Stay-tuned to the blog (www.dataanddonuts.org) for updates on other peripherals and tools...

Clear, concise, authentic

If you want to write well don't look primarily to others for guidance. Many writers have webinars and meetings for quite a fee to lead others into the profession. Throw the rules out of the window. You have a style you have a voice. If you don't like my aversion to inserting "that" in my sentences, find another writer to follow. Think about it. If we all diagram our sentences, follow all the capitalization standards, and become grammar-philes what happens to the agile artistry of putting words on a page? I'm not saying to be lazy. Always be intentional with your writing. I will tell you, the clients hiring you for medical writing (the large majority) are not going to appreciate leaner prose or focused content. They prefer "utilize" and will put it back as fast as you can edit. You won't be given an opportunity to respond line-by-line regarding why you chose this word or that word and how the nuance in one of the edits changes the entire meaning or infrastructure of the document. As a hired gun don't be too precious with your "darlings"--let them edit and wordsmith. They won't be improving the document but they will be happier with the vision they had for the outcome. Hopefully it still resonates with a respectable degree of clarity.

Obviously if you are writing manuscripts you need to follow the more or less strict expectation of "tight" professional writing. You convey a professional, personality free narrative that only communicates the science. I taught science writing and with a few easily applied rules, a strong non-fiction reading habit, and practice--viola, students were ready for work. There are quite a few reliable writing books but I think the most enduring is William Zinger on Writing Well, a great guide for nonfiction writing. Here are easy rules to consider.

Replace utilize with use--simplify your language

Remove the verb "to be"...these are lazy words--challenge yourself to find something better.

-Is

-Are
-Was
-Were
-Be
-Been
-Am

Stop splitting the infinitive (keep subject and main verb close), write in active voice (subject, verb, object) turning verbs into nouns, use strong verbs, and edit out unnecessary words

Social media

"There is no specific platform for being an ass, and you have now found two"

The opening quote was sent to me in response to a discussion on Facebook. Be prepared to be on the receiving end of rude comments from time to time. If you can handle the false bravado of content viewers with an axe to grind I suggest reaching out on social media. The ability to reach a larger audience with minimal effort can create an active bidirectional community. If you develop online content, "best practices" include embracing this quick media tool to drive viewers, clicks, and notability for measured messages and adverts. As a consumer of digital information you can quickly fall into a rabbit hole of pseudoscience as you pursue the immediacy of distilled information.

I am fairly new to blogging. I started Data & Donuts less than 6 months ago. In that time we have had well over 4000 unique visitors to the site and close to 13000 page views. This reflects decent engagement and fulfills my original goal of thoughtful dialogue and discussion in the life of creatives. Here is the rub. Once you begin reaching into the world of social media you are inundated with offers to get to the next milestone--get more readers, more interactions. It begins to resemble a carnival sideshow.

Initially it is quit exciting to watch the impact of new postings, read comments from subscribers, and measure everything you write by its broad applicability and general consumption. Except for one thing. That may not be the reason you blog. I felt and still do that it is important to ask questions. Not necessarily provide solutions but make sure we are all asking the right questions with a healthy dose of skepticism and wonder. A strong empathetic voice rallies attention to a pressing question or an evolving need. The media funnel is 24/7 and in the absence of the ability to think critically--all we have is noise. The listicle in my mind is part of the problem. You know what a listicle describes? Ten ways to increase productivity etc. Someone else is doing the "thinking" and passing along the message. What is wrong with that you might ask? Look at how Google or any search engine is structured. What do you see at the top of any search? Only the latest information. The freshest, most neatly packaged message or topical collection rises to the top. No context, no history, no thought to relevance--just a numbers game.

There aren't any quick fixes for our business or personal challenges. The rise of the "curator of all things" mentality in our digital world seems to dampen our ability to discern what is "meaningful" to what is "here and immediately accessible". Twitter in its most egregious form shouts 140 character sound bites meant to tantalize not necessarily inform. Short cuts in scientific query delude reputable news agencies to pass along dubious research findings. We passively accept the status quo and forget to look with granularity at the actual data. Averages and inferential associations become facts. Commercial interests dilute the common good and warp the true societal need and benefit.

We need to be vigilant and reject the cacophony of the unfiltered. Remain skeptical, and inquisitive. **Keep your eyebrow arched and ask the questions.**

Tips for travel...

I work primarily as a consultant or freelance writer so travel is a necessary business need. Luckily the destinations are typically easily accessible and in actual places I like to visit. This year alone I traveled to meetings in San Diego, New York multiple times, Boston, Philadelphia, Washington DC multiple times, and others are added to the schedule. All things being equal if the train is a viable option I find the opportunity to work while in transit a particularly attractive bonus. Unfortunately that is often coupled with questionable dining choices and the luck of the draw regarding traveling companions but so far, all is well.

Owning a Wi-Fi hotspot or having the ability to connect with your phone's Wi-Fi capabilities is useful when navigating the spotty Internet options on a train in general but Amtrak specifically. I prefer chunking activities into a schedule of reading, editing, and research for the bulk of the trip, and writing once the ducks are aligned.

When traveling to client locations or client specific meetings it is vital to clarify where and when you are expected to attend. Back in the glory days of writing I would regularly be greeted by a limousine driver in the airport and delivered to an address provided by the client. Arriving at my hotel I would unpack, grab a bite to eat, and freshen up before heading to the client site. I remember arriving on site for a meeting, the team was frantic Why wasn't I there for the meeting? Hadn't my flight landed 2 hours ago, blah, blah, blah. The fact that I went where the car was instructed to take me was of no consequence. Always check, recheck, and recheck. Managing expectations whether they are communicated or not is a vital part of freelance work or consultancy. In addition, if you don't want to be the designated person approaching faculty for payment of an apparent hotel porn addiction be certain to have clearly defined onsite responsibilities. Live it and learn it...

An additional lesson that fortunately I never learned the hard way-- travel in professional attire if arriving by airline or any time you will be separated from your luggage during your commute. I heard of a colleague that was forced to moderate a medical meeting in a velour sweat suit. Don't let that be you. I have retired the formal suit in favor of a simple professional dress. Unfortunately I don't see avoiding the suit if you are a man but the ease of travel is exponentially increased if you can roll up a few wrap dresses into a suitcase with a pair of heels and a small bag of jewelry options.

It is advantageous to keep your office humming along in your absence. If you are active on social media I suggest using tools that can be preloaded with content for scheduled postings. I primarily use Edgar, Feedly, or Buffer. It's like having a mini assistant to handle the office in your absence.

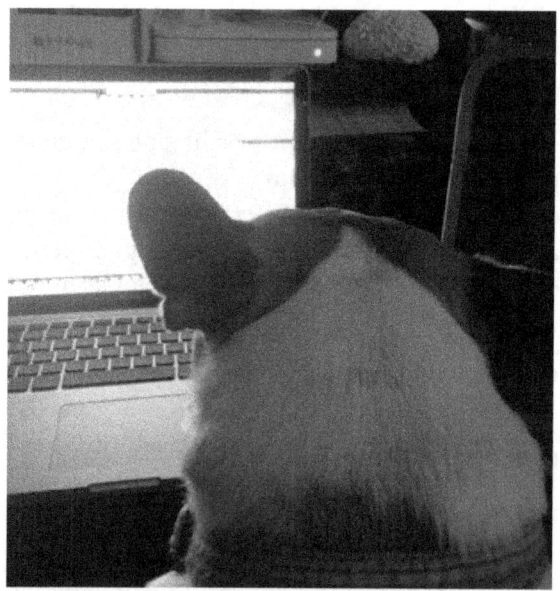

If you are a frazzled traveler and never see the light of day during busy meetings I suggest you find something to pursue in every city. There never seems to be enough time for me to visit every museum collection but I am a champ at the museum gift shop perusal.

Don't be a fungus

You know the type. An all suffering colleague or writing professional too busy to do anything but "work" or paint the illusion of work, waves off opportunities to engage. I begin most days with a run or a workout. Writing is hard work and running a business is hard work. As an employee you are still a self-contained business. Advantages gained by being fit and clear of mind are obvious. I can't tell you how often I have met the CEO, thought leader, or chairman of an event running in the pre-dawn either outside or on the treadmill.

Data insights

It is useful as a medical/science writer to be well versed in data analytics. There are many resources (topic for another book) so here is a brief introduction to freely available tools to explore.

Tableau Public

Full disclosure, Tableau is my visualization tool of choice. It just seems to be a little more intuitive to my non-IT brain although before you know it you might be writing code and finding new business opportunities for your expanding skills. If you can manage simple excel tasks it shouldn't be too difficult to combine those skills and create, collaborate, share interactive charts and graphs, maps, live dashboards and then publish anywhere in your digital space. Tableau Public is free and available online.

As an independent content creator and insight analyst I have invested a few years learning basic coding skills and refreshing my years of statistics. If you too want to be able to use data to inform your content development I think Tableau is the best data visualization tool on the market. The only limitation is a lack of a modeling capability so if you work with HEOR data you still need access to more evolved simulation and modeling tools such as micro-simulation tool for chronic disease modeling (MIST).

Workflows continuously evolve depending on projects or collaborations. The challenge of working with physician experts across a variety of disease states in medical education, healthcare policy, advisory panels, and even monographs or white papers is a much more fluid enterprise and if you have the ability to stay current on a few modest technologic advances you will be rewarded with efficiency and shared success across a variety of evolving platforms.

Plotl.y

Plotly is a tool with a free option powered for collaborative sharing. You have the ability to combine different data sources into a single visualization. Create charts for reports or dashboards and integrate into PowerPoint or email. You may have noticed that a few government datasets allow integration with plotly at just a press of a button!

OpenRefine

Another free resource that evolved over the years was Google Refine. Now, no longer affiliated with Google, and renamed OpenRefine, it is a robust tool with a bit of a learning curve but strong community and online support tools. The real sweet spot for OpenRefine is managing datasets that require cleaning before analysis.

Data freely available to the public

Public-Use Data Files and Documentation

"The National Center for Health Statistics (NCHS) is pleased to offer downloadable public-use data files through the Centers for Disease Control and Prevention's (CDC) FTP file server. Users of this service have access to data sets, documentation, and questionnaires from NCHS surveys and data collection systems. Downloading instructions are available in "readme" files.

Public-use data files are prepared and disseminated to provide access to the full scope of the data. This allows researchers to manipulate the data in a format appropriate for their analyses. NCHS makes every effort to release data collected through its surveys and data systems in a timely manner.

Users of NCHS public-use data files must comply with data use restrictions to ensure that the information will be used solely for statistical analysis or reporting purposes."

Datasets listed on the CDC website include:

National Health Care Surveys

-National Ambulatory Medical Care Survey (NAMCS)

-National Hospital Ambulatory Medical Care Survey (NHAMCS)

-National Hospital Discharge Survey (NHDS)

-National Survey of Ambulatory Surgery (NSAS)

-National Home and Hospice Care Survey (NHHCS)

-National Nursing Home Survey (NNHS)

-National Nursing Assistant Survey (NNAS)

National Vital Statistics Systems

-Vital Statistics Online - Access to downloadable datasets

-Natality (Births)

-Mortality (Deaths)

-Linked Birth/Infant Death

-Fetal Death

-National Mortality Followback Survey (NMFS)

-Matched Multiple Birth Data Set

-Mortality Component - Instruction Manuals

-MICAR Data Dictionary

National Health Interview Survey

-Questionnaires, Datasets, and Related Documentation

National Immunization Survey (NIS)

-Public-Use Data Files

Longitudinal Studies of Aging (LSOA)

Why data matters…

Let's use an example of mammograms' effectiveness to detect breast cancer. Not to be too simplistic but let's consider how we might gather the necessary statistics. If we identify a positive mammogram what is the probability that we indeed detected cancer?

According to the publically available American Cancer Society there are about 231,840 new cases of invasive breast cancer detected each year. Each year there are 38,770,390 mammographies performed. Since the accuracy of mammograms varies from 80% to 90% let's assume 90% for purposes of calculations. By adding the 10% of false positives to the estimated 231, 840 cases per year we have the probability of a positive mammogram indicating breast cancer to be 231,840/4108879 or roughly about 5%.

The cost of US mammograms vary from $100 with a reported average of $243 reported by a copay data aggregator, so those 38,770,390 mammograms cost about 3.8 billion dollars if we are using the low cost range. Each case of breast cancer would cost about $18000 to diagnose and that does not even account for the biopsy required for confirmation that would likely double the 3.8 billion figure to above 7 billion yielding $34,000 dollars for the average cost of initial diagnosis.

One more step here. Since only one out of every 2000 women screened will have their life extended--if 38,770,390 women are screened each year that means that 19,385 women will have their lives extended by early screening to the cost of $361,103 per mammogram. This figure does not include treatment costs or other indirect costs related to the lives extended each year due to screenings.

Go find the data that is meaningful to you!

Where are the clients?

Jay Z said it best. I am a business. Man. (or woman) I am surprised how many freelance types don't consider themselves a business. I find the word "freelance" limiting but for ease of level setting it describes the gist of what it means to create content (or any other creative endeavor) for hire. I put on my consultant hat when there is a time specific project that requires integration across teams or business objectives.

Clients are interested in my strategic perspective on let's say a grander scale when I am brought in as a consultant. For example, as a freelancer I may be asked to perform a network meta-analysis on a certain subset of clinical trial data. When brought in as a consultant I would be advising on the appropriate data strategy and statistical analytics, collaborating with the statistical team, providing oversight, and writing a report or article for publication.

Entrepreneur is another differentiating term that indicates a certain autonomic capacity to generate income. As an author for example, I can generate income even when I am not actively working on a project. Digital access to my growing portfolio means that the "business" is open 24/7. If you want to blog, create unique content, or develop branded content you are also a business. Your voice is as unique as your fingerprints. What we like, our pursuits, environment, and most of all our character inform us. Think about what three words might describe your product. You might discover a winning and marketable brand with a waiting market!

The majority of clients that I engage find me on LinkedIn. If you don't have a dynamic and frequently updated profile I would start there. *Go ahead. I'll wait.* Many experts provide bulleted lists of specific actions to increase your profile traffic but I think it is more important to be consistent with your personality, culture, and brand. The only absolutes are to have a nice photo and engaging content on your profile page. Writing published posts, contributing to or developing a group, and being active on the platform will definitely increase your exposure.

No matter what paid courses and publications will promise there are no secrets to landing long-term, high paying clients. Create a platform unique to you where you can grow your profile. First be of service. Your clients aren't necessarily looking for a freelance writer or analyst. They have a problem that needs solving. You might be the solution...

Your DNA is 99.9% the same as everyone else's. The tiny .1% that is different, is your distinct value.--Sally Hogshead

Bonus: Where to find the data

Here is the opportunity as I see it. Innovative advances in medicine and healthcare delivery are being made each and every day. The final delivery of that care is the real determinant as to whether an intervention is successful. While technology and innovation is important what we really need is process innovation. We need to deliver the right care to the right people in the right time frame and right sequence.

The electronic health record (EHR)/electronic medical record (EMR) system is integrated into daily practice on an escalating basis so lets achieve the vision promised by information technology. Financial costs continue to be aggregated and analyzed at the specialty or service department level. What we need to do is focus on the costs of treating patients over their full cycle of care. Let's stop measuring the wrong things the wrong way...

Data is everywhere and it seems that everyone has a handle on this new source of useable information—but do they? In healthcare especially much of the data is behind a firewall, proprietary and/or access is monetized as part of a business model or opportunity. Perhaps there are glimpses here and there visible at conferences or embedded in news articles but what do you do if you would like to analyze your own data?

Unless you have deep pockets and can afford the industry data access it isn't likely you want to spend thousands and thousands of dollars to access IMS data, a leader in the billion-dollar pharmaceutical data industry. I observed my bookshelf and although I have quite a few books about healthcare data I rely on only a chapter here and there from each book. That is where the idea for short chapter books specific to a business need was generated. I curated the most frequent questions from my blog and created a publication strategy for short topics as an introduction and a quick how-to resource. This format is also easily updated and can be integrated into a curated series based on your own level and interests.

Let's see where we can find some useful data for our proposals, websites, corporate blogs, brand content, and digital communication strategies.

Patient Level Data

There are a variety of sources of longitudinal patient data (LPD). The data is de-identified and can be collected from health claims data, pharmacy records, electronic medical records, and any other source that tracks data linearly over a period of time.

What type of information can you potentially derive from patient level data?

Prevalence and incidence, demographics, treatment protocols, patient referrals, prescriptions, days on treatment, sequence of drug regimens, screening, vaccinations, adherence, are just a few examples of the type of data available. I have extensive experience analyzing electronic medical record data useful for measuring how specific drugs are being prescribed and by whom, what are the dosages, how have prescribing trends shifted over time (are they influenced by sampling for example), what percentage of patient population is comorbid, treatment sequence data--the granularity of new, switch, add-on, etc. dynamics are also relevant. Why are patients switching? What are the outcomes on the new regimens?

The value of including this type of data in content documents or reporting is measuring actual prescribing and patient management data in real time. Patient-level data removes the bias inherent in survey instruments and allows deeper dives into the data. For example, you can evaluate data by indication, line of treatment, market dynamics, and comorbidity.

Industry stakeholders are making claims of value and requesting that brand strategies, continuing educational programs, and digital media advertising integrate a narrative voice. The ability to identify data strategies relevant throughout a product or brand lifecycle can be effective in engaging an audience and facilitating relevant discussion.

Patient data collected over time in a linear manner provides insights during all phases of a product lifecycle. Integrated into a needs assessment to contextualize a perceived gap in clinical care or to determine efficacy or evaluation of market strengths and/or weaknesses collected prior to launch establishes identification of facilitators or barriers to uptake. In addition, the ability to stratify data by cohorts may be useful in identifying clinical trial participants, create meaningful endpoints, and create a value proposition.

Assets moving into phase III benefit from positioning data relevant for pricing strategies and value statement refinement prior to commercialization and identification for targeting, messaging, and promotion. Research and Development (R&D) launch is no longer the end-post. Market access is optimized by observational studies demonstrating real world evidence and multiple sources of data are needed to continuously adjust value messaging in the shifting landscape of new and emergent therapies. Additional data is needed as patents expire and generic formulations require efficacy and safety messages.

Data of Interest to Industry and Physicians

There have been influential posts in social media successful at creating awareness around abusive trends in Medicare payments to providers. The source of the data has been in part the transparency required by provisions in the Affordable Care Act. The ability to drill into reimbursement data at the regional, provider, and therapeutic level is instrumental in identifying potential sources of inefficiencies and spiraling costs.

Datasets are updated and released periodically by Centers for Medicare & Medicaid Services (CMS) and include payments made directly, indirectly or by third party payers. In addition an integrated search tool and Data Exchange Tool allows access to visualize and analyze datasets or to download a full dataset. The views available include data lens, datasets, charts, maps, calendars, filtered views, external datasets, forms, and even APIs.

> **"With Data Lens, governments can finally shift from simple, data-centric citizen interaction to an information-centric experience. Government data becomes dramatically more accessible and impactful for citizens, community advocates, journalists, and employees."**

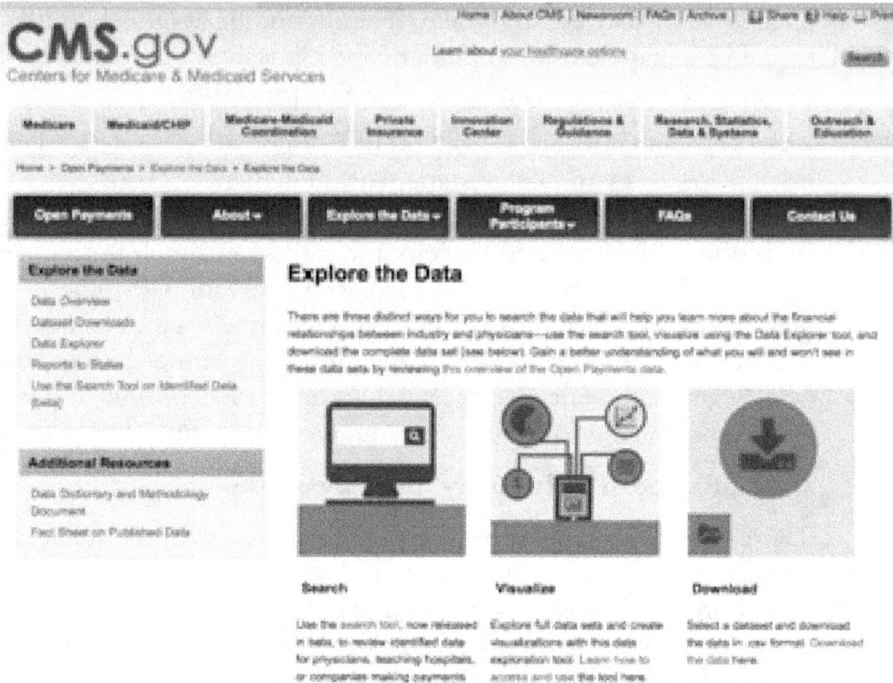

Data of Interest for Providers and Consumers

Clinicaltrial.gov is a useful "web-based resource that provides patients, their family members, health care professionals, researchers, and the public with easy access to information on publicly and privately supported clinical studies on a wide range of diseases and conditions".

The National Library of Medicine (NLM) at the National Institutes of Health (NIH) includes information updated by the sponsor or principal investigator of the clinical study. At specific points during the longitudinal timeline or often submitted after the study ends, data is uploaded to the site. This database of clinical studies is a "registry" and "results database."

Graphics are often available for inclusion in reports or content media platforms as well as downloads for content analysis. I have included a few data visualization tools that (in addition to Excel) are useful in preparing data for analyses.

Of particular interest for health policy content paramount in the expansion of the site or highlighting specific influencers of market access in cancer research is the History, Policy, and Laws link, https://clinicaltrial.gov/ct2/about-site/history.

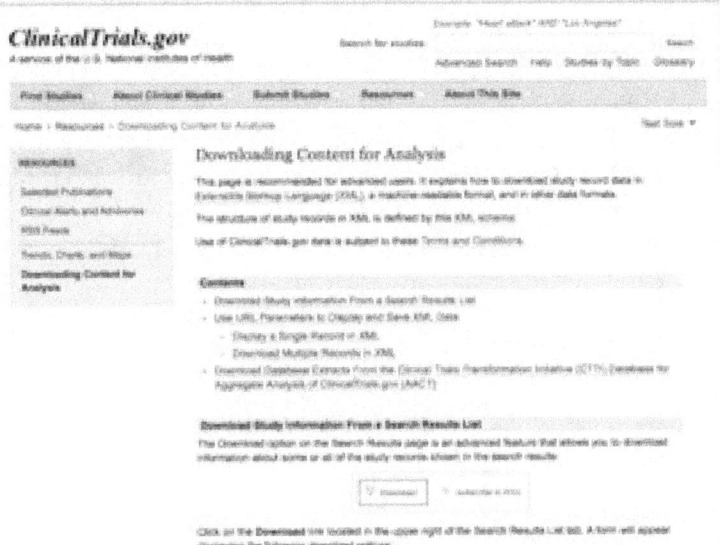

The Agency for Healthcare Research and Quality (AHRQ) hosts the HCUPnet, a free, on-line query system based on data from the Healthcare Cost and Utilization Project (HCUP). It provides access to health statistics and information on hospital inpatient and emergency department utilization and State Emergency Department Databases for emergency department (ED) visits that do not result in hospitalizations.

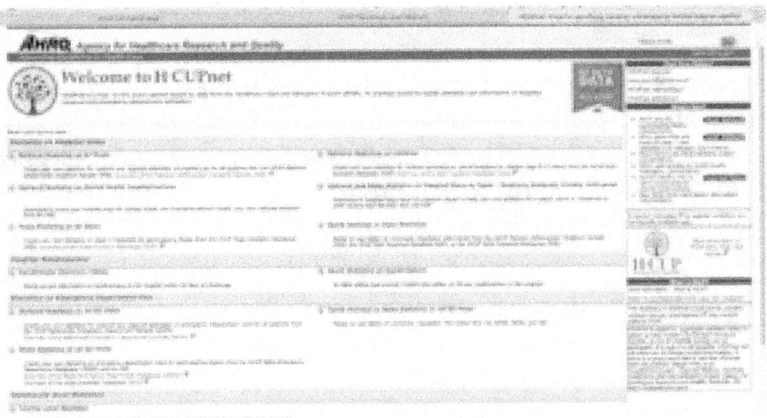

Data of Interest to Providers and Community

Data.gov links to over 245 state and federal healthcare datasets such as hospital charge data that can be searched by diagnosis-related groups (DRG)-- a system to classify hospital cases into specific groups, Agency for Healthcare Research and Quality (AHRQ), community healthcare centers, and Veterans Affairs data, for example. The screencast below lists a specific DRG and average and total payments for covered charges and Medicare payments. Visualization options are also listed in the expanded right column in addition options to export data for analyses, or filter by region for example.

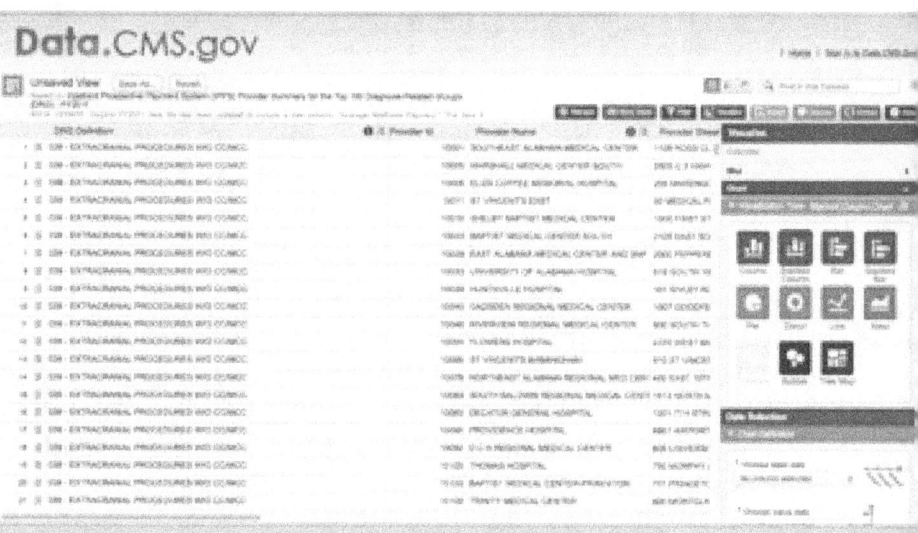

The Surveillance, Epidemiology, and End Results (SEER) Program of the National Cancer Institute provides cancer statistics to help reduce the burden of cancer within the U.S. Released every spring with updated data from the prior November's submission date, the website currently includes 18 SEER registries from different years of diagnoses based on enrollment in the SEER program.

There are several interactive tools providing data access to answer a variety of health economics and clinical awareness questions. The ability to provide context for funding requests, awareness, or even brand positioning relies on a strong data informed narrative. A variety of linked data sources are available for review and analyses.

Data of Interest to Provider, Consumer, Community

Healthdata.gov is a one-stop portal for free, publicly available data. Disease specific national and regional data is reported by CMS, Centers for Disease Control, Department of Health and Human Services in addition to state agencies, that cover over 1900 datasets. Health Data Initiative Starter Kit provides an introduction overview to the types of data linked on the site.

I hope that you learned about a few new resources to help integrate data informed content for your medical communication objectives.

Getting started

"Statistics are like swimwear - what they reveal is suggestive but what they conceal is vital." -Ashish Mahajan, Lancet 2007

Don't forget to add basic statistic skills to your toolbox. You need at minimum the ability to navigate research publications and distinguish between low-value and high-value evidence.

This deserves repeating. If you automate as much of your business infrastructure as possible, your day is ready. I typically work on a few blogs and then settle into client work. The ebb and flow is manageable and I find myself lucky to pursue high-value work. Integrating economics, health policy, and clinical medicine into a compelling narrative isn't a bad way to spend your work life. Freelance work is not for everyone. If you crave independence and meaningful work I encourage you to give it a try--swimsuit optional.

Here is a list of a few of my favorite time savers:

Feedly (filter RSS fields of interest into one source)

Buffer (schedule social media posts around a variety of time zones)

Canva (add a design flare to images)

Sumo (free tools to simplify your website/blog)

Weebly (the best platform for my website/blog)

Atavist (you worry about the content, Atavist will take care of everything else)

iTunes (podcasts) for finding your "thinky" thoughts

Public Library (e-books)

Storify (for a quick search for what everyone is talking about)

Mail Chimp (best way to keep in touch with your "tribe" through quick easy newsletters)

Once you write a few stories in the public domain you can apply for membership to the Association of Health Care Journalists. Unparalleled access to a variety of resources is one of the advantages of joining. I am fluid about my American Medical Writing Association membership. It really isn't something I miss when I lapse but as an organization I like to support their efforts. Perhaps you want to take a course or a certification? They might be a good resource but in the age of Coursera and other massive open online courses (MOOCs) you might find better courses for free. Lynda.com is another quick skill resource if you need to brush up on a little coding or social media skills. Although not free, the nominal fee is worth always having access to a variety of useful business skills.

No need to reinvent the wheel. These are useful frameworks for you to apply to your content strategy. Don't hesitate to customize and find your own short cuts. But most of all...read!

A Case Study

I would like to encourage a critical eye and curiosity to dig a little deeper in matters of medical content writing. This example has broad applicability to all channels of writing. A 2012 article by Mills and colleagues discusses How to Use an Article Reporting a Multiple Treatment Comparison Meta-Analysis (JAMA, September 26, 2012—Vol 308, No 12). I stumbled across the paper as a resource for a network meta-analysis report that I am writing so I thought it might be interesting to apply the rigor and granularity to developing a framework for medical education assessment.

A clinical scenario describing a 45-year old patient prescribed a selective serotonin reuptake inhibitor (SSRI) 6 weeks prior to treat generalized anxiety disorder (GAD) is typical of question stems presented to measure physician competence or practice behavior. She is being seen in your office today reporting improved symptoms but now states that she has insomnia and a reduced interest in sex. The task for your outcomes team is to find out how to assess the appropriate care of this patient in a medical education intervention. How can you compare treatments that reflect the clinical considerations of a busy physician practice? I review the questions during program analyses and cringe at the treatment options included in the educational assessment. Understanding that patient management is not akin to baking a cake there are no inherently wrong or right answers. Patient centric behavior included the perspective of what provides "value" and quality of life (QOL) to each individual patient. When outcomes teams select old standard of care, inferior therapies with significant adverse event profiles as options in an assessment learning is not going to happen.

You might be tempted to list a few other drugs randomly with an indication for GAD but how can we dig a little deeper and display an appropriate algorithm for evaluating multiple efficacy and safety data from all drugs available to treat patients with GAD. We need to research multiple treatment comparison (MTC) meta-analyses for the opportunity to include head-to-head randomized clinical trial evidence

(RTC) and indirect evidence to evaluate all of the available interventions. A clinician in a practice environment will be obtaining specific information from the patient that will require a fluid understanding of research findings and a comparative model to review evidentiary findings across the available evidence-based research.

Evidence-based recommendations rely on randomized controlled trials (RCT) to arrive at treatment recommendations in healthcare decisions. The comparators in many of these trials vary and are often placebo, older standard of care or another comparator to placebo but quite often not direct treatment comparisons. Non-inferiority studies also lack the ability to identify the optimal drug in any algorithm. These indirect comparisons are not without their merit and understanding how to interpret evidence across competing interventions to select appropriate treatments is critical. Network meta-analyses provide estimates for effect sizes calculated regardless of whether they are direct or indirect.

Critical appraisal of a network meta-analysis requires assessment of the clinical trial characteristics.

Are the studies, outcomes, design, and populations similar for comparison?

Critical Appraisal Guide to a Multiple Treatment Comparison— *from User Guides to The Medical Literature*

Meta-analysis—quick checklist for review

A. Are the results of the study valid?

Did the review explicitly address a sensible clinical question?

Was the search for relevant studies exhaustive?

Were there major biases in the primary studies?

B. What are the results?

What was the amount of evidence in the network?

Were the results similar from study to study?

Were the results consistent in direct and indirect comparisons?

What were the overall treatment effects and their uncertainty, and how did the

treatments rank?

Were the results robust to sensitivity assumptions and potential biases?

C. How can I apply the results to patient care?

Were all patient-important outcomes considered?

Were all potential treatment options considered?

Are any postulated subgroup effects credible?

What is the overall quality and what are limitations of the evidence?

These evaluations are critical to reveal the quality of evidence informing treatment decisions at the point of care. Determining low-value or high-value inferences should guide treatment decisions to alternative options with improved tolerability.

fine

About the Author

Transitioning early in her career as a chiropractor working with pediatric patients to a bench scientist in population genetics, Bonny has worked in academia/medicine, industry, and medical education in many therapeutic areas. As a medical writer her responsibilities and skills evolved into executive roles within medical education and a career developing analytical insights and actionable data-driven recommendations into content media, industry reports and powerful market access documentation. In addition to integrating value strategy in alignment with business development activities Bonny joins collaborative teams with an active role creating strategies and tactics for economic value and quality of life arguments during development, launch, and lifecycle management. Ongoing academic work in model thinking, discrete choice experiments, and health technology assessment has created a variety of opportunities to improve patient outcomes at the point of care. Bonny is also working with the Right Care Alliance to advocate for the health needs of patients and communities to invest in the policies and infrastructure that best serve the interests of community. https://www.dataanddonuts.org

Other books by this author

Please visit your favorite ebook retailer to discover other books by Bonny P McClain

5 Sources for the Right Healthcare Data: Bigger isn't Always Better

Connect with Bonny McClain

I really appreciate you reading my book! Here are my social media coordinates:

Friend me on Facebook: http://facebook.com/dataanddonuts

Follow me on Twitter: https://twitter.com/graphemeconsult

Favorite my Amazon author page: http://www.amazon.com/author/bonnymcclain

Subscribe to my blog: http://www.dataanddonuts.org

Connect on LinkedIn: https://www.linkedin.com/in/bonnypmcclain

Visit my website: http://www.dataanddonuts.org/what-we-do.html

www.ingramcontent.com/pod-product-compliance
Lightning Source LLC
Chambersburg PA
CBHW070922180526
45168CB00005B/2119